THE BEST SUCCESS IS HAPPINESS

Debbie Loane

A route to living a happy and fulfilling life

The path we are on is not the only one.
We can change direction with our thoughts.

We are the creators of our own reality.
We are responsible for our own lives.
All we need is within us. Focusing within ourselves
is the way to a fulfilling life.

The beliefs we hold determine our success or failure.
We inherit beliefs about ourselves and the world as we live.

--------   --------------

Expect the best. That is what we deserve. We can decide
how our reality will be and create that reality.

The relationship with ourselves must come first.
Self love is the starting point to sharing love.

Love is the universal connection.
We come here to live in love.

The path we are on is not the only one.

We can change direction with our thoughts.

This book started through journaling, not a daily account of life. But more writing thoughts and ideas to figure what are the components of living a complete, conscious, satisfying life. Trying to figure and give thought to, what it's all about, why are we here, what it is important to achieve, how we all differ and are we all connected within a universal power or energy? The title gives an indication as to the subject. The readers may ask, do I have a qualification to write about this subject? Have I been taught by a guru, taken courses in relevant subjects? The answer is no! This book is not based on what I've been taught although, I have read many good books and watched videos on this and related subjects for leisure and my interest in getting the most from life and living it to the full. Trying to understand why, for many people life seems difficult and unhappy and for others it seems to flow without much effort. My interest was first sparked by a correspondence life coach diploma course. I completed it a number of years ago. It was when most life coaching was done in one-to-one, face-to-face sessions. Helping the client to work through life situations and 'seeing the wood for the trees 'so to speak.

I did that course simply for the enjoyment of it. The assignments were easy for me to complete. I found it interesting and enjoyable. I have an incredibly logical outlook on life which on numerous occasions has been identified by others. Maybe it's not something that serves well in all situations. But when problems arise and people focus on all the outer fluff of the situation and get tied up in the nitty gritty, I can generally put things in perspective, identify the core of what is happening and name it.

This is a book from personal experience. My thinking has changed and now at 60 years old I feel like I had been living unconsciously for years but then slowly gave thought to how things were and realised that I was in charge of how my life unfolded. The biggest part being that our mind and our reality are a direct result of our thoughts. So I'm writing this for the reader who, perhaps hasn't considered how our thinking directly effects our feelings, our outlook, and our day to day lives, ultimately how happy we feel. Maybe then can give consideration to and gain awareness of their thoughts, and realise how this can change their reality. What goes on in our minds both consciously and subconsciously is what makes the ultimate difference to the kind of life we experience. Our thoughts shape our day to day lives. There are numerous books written on the subject of how to improve our lives. This one is perhaps best for the reader who is starting their journey of self discovery and becoming aware of the connection between body and mind and the connection between the individual and the collective universal energy.

Everyone's ultimate goal one would assume is to be happy. To live life feeling happy and contented day to day. Unfortunately for many people they look outside themselves to obtain happiness. Usually blaming others or outside circumstances for the unhappiness they encounter in their lives. I am now aware that happiness comes from within. This awareness and the changes I have made in my life since changing my thoughts are responsible for the happy life I now enjoy. We are responsible for our own happiness. So the good news is that no matter how terrible we consider our lives to be, we are the ones with the power to change it. By changing our thoughts and mindset it is possible to experience a different reality. The one we choose hour to hour and day by day, can over time become the mindset which can create the life we choose.

This book has come about from my realisation, awareness, and what I've experienced in my life. In many ways the experiences and subjects that I write about seem logical, basic ideas that I would have assumed are widespread common knowledge. But since I have become aware of this conscious thinking and living, I realise that it's not common place. I have not studied or done a life's work of research. But once I gave time and thought and developed an interest in how we create our reality, I became aware of how simple steps can change our thinking. These concepts are easy to understand and to execute. My goal is that the reader gains awareness and can put these into practice in their own life. The challenges we deal with in life will not change but how we deal with them will make a difference to our experiences.

We are the creators of our own reality.
We are responsible for our own lives.
All we need is within us. Focusing within
ourselves is the way to a fulfilling life.

Are you aware of the voice in your head? The near constant chatter that takes place in your mind. I'm not sure when I became aware of it. I think like most people you know it's there but don't really acknowledge what a major part of your life it is. Unless you really become aware of it, think about it and start to monitor what it is saying, it can be one of the most destructive things in your life. However, alternatively it can be beneficial with awareness. Considering it's that life altering, I wonder how it took me so long before I really took notice of it. I suspect other people are the same or perhaps go their whole lives without being fully aware of its relevance and how it can constantly effect their lives. If we observe it for a while, we can see if it is something of benefit or destruction. Unfortunately in the majority of people without an awareness of it, it tends to be a destructive force they constantly live with.

Consider the amount of time everyday that the voice is chattering away in your head. In every scenario that happens or most likely doesn't happen, the voice is at work. Preempting scenarios, preempting responses and the unfortunate thing is that in most cases it's preempting things you don't actually want to happen. So you take something that you don't want to occur in your life and you give it life.

You imagine the problem, the worry, the hassle, the loss, whatever it is, you build a picture. You start a conversation telling yourself how it will go. If there is another person in the scenario, which there often is, you conduct this two way conversation playing both parts yourself. On it goes, sometimes for hours or even days. Perhaps the scenario does come to pass. Maybe not as you imagined, or perhaps it does not happen at all. But you have spent the time preempting and imagining a life event or scenario, which when you were giving it your full attention and living it in your head did not exist. It was a made up scenario with a dialogue. It was something that you thought had the possibility of being part of your future. But future events are not real. The only place future events can take place are in our minds. So the whole scenario, which a conversation has taken place about back and forth, possibly arguing your point, trying to convince another to see your point of view, trying to convince them they are mistaken, perhaps trying to convince them to help you in some way. The only place this conversation is real is in your head. It's not real anywhere else or for anyone else. It's not even real for you because it's not happening at that time. It's not real it's just in your head.

This is exactly how we bring stress into our lives. It starts ao imagined events or scenarios. We go with all the what ifs, that might occur and we build them up. Not only during the day as we go about our lives but often in bed, lying awake our thoughts start. Creating one negative scenario after the next. We can lie awake and create all sorts of worrying thoughts which can mushroom and rob us of our sleep. The feeling associated with negative thinking is stress. We create and experience it. But at the time we are experiencing these feelings of stress, the event is not real, only imagined in our minds. So it can not be solved. It is a useless exercise. Although a very common one. The stress that's experienced is destructive and can cause an effect both mentally and physically.

When we read it like that and we give consideration to all the events that play out in our mind, the conversations that are conducted there, the arguments we have, the disagreements, the worries, the illness, the fears, the loss, the suffering, we become aware that none of this is real. We are creating the entire thing in our mind. It is not part of our reality at that time and may never be part of our reality.

We could argue that by preempting what is likely to happen

in the future and trying to deal with it and take precautions, we are being sensible and perhaps averting a crisis. Well that is perhaps true. But in this situation we are taking action in the present moment. Putting in work, making plans, preparing, perhaps studying. Doing something which we consider might benefit our future. This is a different thing than dealing with a perceived future event in our head. Playing out a scenario in our head of a presumed future event won't effect the outcome, if the situation does occur in the future. It can't effect it because it is not real at that moment, only imagined. Past events can bring similar feelings of stress into our lives as we relive it, analyzing what happened, what was said, how we felt. What could have been different. But as with future events, they cannot be changed in the now moment.

Unfortunately when we run things over and over in our minds it's usually negative things in our life. Negative thoughts are much more prevalent. If we experience a positive event and recall it, it probably puts a smile on our face as we do. It gives us a nice feeling. We conjure up a picture perhaps. It's a good experience! The likelihood is it might enter our head again in the future. Might cause us to smile again but in general it is not to the forefront of our mind for long. If our mind goes from one thought to the next with thought association, it will stay on a positive trail of the good memories associated with it. Which will induce positive feelings.

Negativity seems to be different. Events which have us feeling negative such as past hurts, disappointments, arguments, whether dealt with to our satisfaction or not, can be recalled over and over, analyzed and given various outcomes in our mind. Past negative events or perceived future events can offer immense fuel to keep a dialogue going in our mind over and over. By giving our attention to future negative scenarios, we may in fact bring them into being. What we give our thoughts to we can create in our life. It is possible through the feelings of stress and worry that are invoked by thoughts, to attract negativity into our lives. It is happening in the mind but has an effect on our whole being.

Do you recognize these types of thoughts .

1 I'm not doing overtime this week. I don't care how busy it is in the office. I did it the last two weeks. Mary gets away with the excuse of her sick mother. I bet she doesn't go visit her half as much as she says. Maybe I'll say Rose is doing revision for exams this week and asked me to come straight home to help." No" I won't say that. I've done my share. If they would stop chatting and having cigarette breaks, we wouldn't need to do so much overtime. It's not worth it after tax. Maybe during the afternoon I'll say I'm not feeling too well. Or I've a ticket for something. No they'll only ask too many questions about where I'm going and with whom. I'm just not doing it. If Mary can say no, so can I. It's not fair. On and on it goes, this pointless conversation in our minds about something which at that moment is only real in the mind.

2 I wonder what Mary really meant when she said my outfit had a lovely casual vibe. The others were probably more dressy. Maybe she was trying to say I wasn't dressy enough for the occasion. Although her own shoes looked a bit worn. Maybe my dress was a bit tight. I should have worn the other one. But this one, casual as she called it, didn't have a casual price tag. I think it cost nearly two weeks wages. Although I have it a while, maybe I look too old for it now. Mutton dressed as lamb. I'm not wearing that anymore. Bit of a nerve commenting on it, not as if she looked fabulous. Ah, she did look well if I'm honest. They all did, I suppose. Maybe if I lost some weight. It looked a bit tight I think, it must be the weight, too tight. On and on it goes, round and round in our minds!

3 Maybe I shouldn't have bought those tickets. Since reading about how many people are sick with flu. If either of us get it we won't get our money back. Oh I'll go mad if I lose that money. They were expensive tickets. He was coughing last night, hope that's not the first sign. Apparently Mary's mum has it. If Mary gets it I won't have a babysitter. Who else could I get to watch the kids? Don't think the tickets sold out. So I won't be able to resell them either. If the flu is as rampant as they say at the moment, lots of people will be affected. There could be loads of tickets for sale. I shouldn't have bought them. Maybe it's a mistake to have Mary babysitting anyway if her mother has it. I was looking forward to going. But I don't think it's worth the hassle, not knowing what will happen. The two of us could be in bed with flu and the tickets wasted, money gone. But then we might be ok. I'll see if he's still coughing tonight. Wonder should I ring Mary see how she feels. Or maybe Jane and Tom want the tickets. Oh no, if I ask them they might think I'm giving them as a present. I'll check the news later, see if the flu numbers in the hospitals have got any worse. On and on it goes round and round in the thoughts and mind!

When we read these internal conversations like this, it's easy to see how nonproductive these kind of conversations are. But we all have the voice in our head. If we are not aware of it and monitor what it is doing, these type of scenarios go on a great deal of the time. Unchecked they lead from one thought to the next creating a dialogue of situations that cause unease and stress. They are serving us no benefit. They are in fact destructive to us.

All these scenarios were negative situations the thinker did not want in their life. They are incidents one could argue that are part of life whether wanted or not. When the dialogue was taking place the situation was not taking place and in some cases perhaps was never going to. So at that point it was a past or future or maybe never scenario. Things in the past future or maybe, cannot be solved or altered in the now. In the now, they are not real. But thoughts conjure up feelings. They produce negative feelings of stress, panic, or anger which are not the result of any incident actually happening. Numerous conversations in our minds don't come to pass in reality or in some cases wouldn't come to pass except for the focused attention that we give them in our thoughts.

We can get a feeling when we read these scenarios of the stress, negativity, panic and upset that the thinker is inducing as these conversations go on in the mind. Inducing a range of negativity needlessly into their life. Creating feelings of stress which would go with these scenarios although the situation is not happening at the time. The feelings are real and being experienced by the thinker. Stress is mental anguish, worry and anxiety which can trigger hormones that produce a physical reaction in the body over time. This seems to the present logical mind a useless and destructive behavior. But all day, everyday this is the human condition. If we do not become aware of it, it continues and continues to be a very destructive force in our lives.

I remember when I was growing up, my mother spoke about how she was a worrier. Like it was something to be proud of. She wore it like a badge of honor! In fact she accused my dad of not worrying about anything. Which made it sound like she had to shoulder all the family worry and somehow he wasn't doing his share. Dad usually made light of it and turned it into something of a joke. But it was regularly brought up by mum. Apparently she felt she had inherited it from her mum who was also the family worrier. I didn't give much thought to it back then. But with an awareness now of how destructive worrying is, I find it quite amazing. I'm sure many people feel the same as my mum. That they are doing a service to their family by shouldering all the worry for them! I'm also not surprised that it was something she felt she inherited from her mum. We all carry around a lot of learned or inherited beliefs with us through life, accepting them as truth and they may be beliefs that are not serving us well. But we never question them. Mum probably heard her mother speak at times about being a worrier and if like mum, she spoke of it with pride as if she was doing a service for others, mum took this as a belief and something she should accomplish to be of assistance to aid herself and others in life. It's so common to hear people say, I'm really worried about this or that, or this person's situation and in many cases it sounds like they believe they are somehow offering something genuinely good to the person they are speaking of. Worrying about what might happen is an utter waste of time for everyone. It servoe no purpose and changes no situation for the better. EVER !

When you consider what my mum was actually doing, she was figuring every possible scenario that might go wrong with a family member. Giving her attention to it, looking at it for all the possibilities of a solution. Willing these things not to be a reality but bringing the negative feeling that would be associated with them, feelings of panic, stress and anxiety into her life. Although the majority of these incidents probably didn't come to pass, if some did, there is a possibility the attention she gave to them is what assisted them in becoming a reality.

When you become aware of the amount of negative chatter, not only done internally in ones own mind but also in conversations between people, it is incredible the amount of conversations that take place about things we don't want in our lives. Financial lack, illness, global disasters are the most common ones. These are usually mentioned every day in most of the media. But also incidental ones like traffic jams, bad weather and household chores. We spend so much time bringing these into our minds when they are not part of the now moment we have to enjoy.

I recently listened to a radio station doing a vox pop on the streets of a city. People were asked the question "are you concerned about flu this winter, since the hospitals here are facing overcrowding problems? " Shockingly the majority of people answered yes, it was a concern. They had considered it and what it might mean if they got a bad flu.

When we listen to this type of thing on the radio, it would generally make us ask ourselves the question if we hadn't already and provoke feelings associated to our answer. If the radio station had worded the question, "are you filling your thoughts while feeling fit and healthy with concern for an illness which is not guaranteed". Doesn't that sound so different? But I suppose that's not the way we would word a question because in general it's not how we think. It is much more common to see the problem which may affect us. But it would be interesting to hear the response if worded differently. As it was, not one person answered "why would I be concerned about something that is not affecting me?" These people were going about their business in a fit state. The concern about their health was unnecessarily being brought to their attention and into their thoughts. If it was something which they hadn't yet considered, it was now being put into their subconscious mind and their thoughts, and present moment. We consider so many problems which might affect us. There seems to always be potential problems available if we choose to assign them to our lives. But if we can stay present the majority of these perceived problems won't effect our lives.

I was at a point where I was feeling our minds are so

intrinsic to our happiness and how we live our lives that this is huge. It should be taught in school or made so widespread that it is passed from parent to child. It is a very good lesson in how to live life if it could be available to children as they grow up . But after listening to this short clip on the radio and the majority of daily news, I realize how far we are from this being a part of people's awareness. So much negativity is suggested to us each day and we absorb it without any kind of filter and it remains in our subconscious or our thoughts and becomes a part of our life by the feelings it invokes. The role of the subconscious mind is to keep us safe and so it stores information and feelings. What goes in is dealt with as reality in our subconscious. It does not differentiate between feelings from real events and feelings we induce by events which are taking place only in our minds. Everything we consciously or subconsciously absorb has an affect on our feelings. Our feelings are the monitor of our reality. Being conscious of our daily intake of information through media or conversations is taking responsibility for the reality we experience.

So much time is spent with minds full of what the future might hold causing us to worry about all the disasters that might unfold. As a result lives are being lived missing out on the present moment. The tasks we are doing and could be taking enjoyment from in that moment are often lost. Even when we gain awareness of this, it still happens. It seems to be a natural part of the human condition. We are not present a lot of the time. But awareness is the first step in changing our thought pattern.

We spend our present time with our minds in the past or the future. Unfortunately very often with negative scenarios taking place in our minds. Whatever we are doing our mind wanders off from the present task and often to something that is not a pleasant thought. From one thought to the

next a whole scenario is taking place in our m'
result that the task in hand which could hav'
and enjoyable is totally lost. When the min
it, there is often no recollection of what took ̖
present moment. One can drive for miles and see
of the road or scenery. Or cook a meal with no recolle
of adding the ingredients if it's a familiar recipe. The resun
is the present moment is being completely lost and often
replaced by thoughts which are not pleasant or real and are
the cause of stress in our lives.

The awareness of missing out on the present is not in itself
a quick fix. But it can be a start to changing our thinking
over time. Initially we realise that a large part of the present
time is being missed. When the mind wanders to this type
of thinking we can start to recognise it. Stop the thought,
focus attention back to the present moment and what is
being done at the time and give that our full attention. Or
we can stop what we are doing and focus on clearing our
mind of thoughts, be present for a few minutes to clear the
mind and then return to the task in hand. (Meditation and
mindfulness, which is covered later in the book, are the
perfect tools to help with this).

Recognizing that our mind is wandering off, acknowledging
what the thoughts are and moving back to the present
is beneficial to stop us going on with negative thoughts.
These can balloon in our mind and lead on from one thing
to another by thought association. Stopping for a moment
and considering " what are these thoughts, are they serving
us in anyway"? Then deciding to let them go and bring our
mind to the present or some positive thoughts that induce
good feelings. The ultimate goal of course is to become
present as much of the time as possible and enjoy the
present moment, focusing on what is occurring at that time.
Then the feelings we are experiencing are a direct result
of our actions. Like most things the more we practices the

it becomes, but every time we can return our mind to present is benifital.

The reward is that we are not bringing worry, fear, stress and upset, into our life unnecessarily by constantly running an internal negative chatter in our mind. The less time spent with our mind in the past or future the happier our lives will be.

I have found that if there is something on my mind, perhaps something that is taking place but I am not in a position to do anything about it. Something I have no control over but it slips into my mind again and again without warning, it is often helpful to do something that I enjoy. Spending time in nature is helpful to clear the mind and offers benefits of reducing stress and anxiety. It has the capacity to induce positive feelings and an optimistic outlook. Exercise is also something that offers many health benefits and can change our mood by releasing endorphins within the body. Or another approach is to do something we find enjoyable. A hobby like gardening or sewing, perhaps something that we can give focused attention to that can hold our concentration. Drinking water is great for boosting concentration and mood, it sounds simple but just drinking a cold glass of water slowly and giving our concentration to it, can help us feel better and lower anxiety in the body and mind. Distractions around us like music or mechanical noises can make it difficult to concentrate but the greatest disturbance can be in our own mind. Keeping our mind on the task in hand and really focusing and delving into the enjoyment of it, will help to put the incident or worry at bay for a period. Like most things the more we can practice refocusing our thoughts, the easier it will be in difficult situations.

Many people live busy lives. We can be on the go from morning to evening. So suggesting we monitor our thoughts, perhaps feels like an extra burden in our lives. Consider the type of thoughts we regularly have and check the lists below. The first list is things we are not in control of and as such we cannot change no matter how much its in our mind. The second list are the things we can control in our lives so action in those circumstances can be beneficial.

It is surprising the amount of thoughts that are common place and are on the list of things we have no control over. Is your present time spent on thoughts that are futile? Thoughts induce feelings and feelings are the basis of our happiness. Are your thoughts inducing feelings of happiness or upset and fear?

The things we have no control over.

List 1

> The past
>
> The future
>
> The actions of others
>
> The thoughts and feelings and beliefs of others
>
> Who we are related to
>
> The weather
>
> Natural disasters

These things we cannot change because they are not within our control. Giving our attention to these things is usually a route to frustration and stress within our lives.

The things we do have control over .

List 2

Our boundaries

What we give our energy to

The goals we set for ourselves

How we speak to ourselves

How we handle challenges

Our thoughts and actions

Our response / reaction

The items on this second list, we are each responsible for in our own lives. These are things we do have choices about and can take action and make decisions on.

There are always things in life which we can get annoyed about or offended by. Some people seem to have a radar that can pick one thing after another to complain about, which cause them upset. These people are normally unhappy with the circumstances in their life and project this onto others. We all have at some times found things annoying or frustrating. But with a mindset of acceptance, it is truly possible to react differently to a situation.

I lived in a costal property in a tourist area a few years ago. With the start of the summer season the watersports equipment and jet skis would be put out and available for hire. That brought with it additional noise to the area. I never felt annoyed or offended by this. The result was that unless someone brought it to my attention, I didn't hear it. My neighbor however was not keen on tourists visiting the area. He stood regularly overlooking the beach complaining about the noise. He tried on occasion to get agreement from me about the situation. I told him that for the most part I didn't hear them but I could not convince him that this was the truth. I realised that because we both felt differently about the water sports our experiences were totally different. I had no issue with them. As a result they didn't disturb me. He on the other hand was so against them, that they were all consuming in his mind and so he was constantly aware of the noise. This I'm sure caused him to have negative internal chatter about them regularly. Acceptance of circumstances in life which are out of our control as this was, makes them easier to live with.(he of course had the choice of whether to continue to live at that location). It takes the negativity away when we accept what is beyond our control.

It is hard to imagine being happy all the time. It is not realistic. Like hot and cold, Ying and Yang, to know one you must know the other. But the overall principle of keeping our minds in the present is certainly a way to avoid upset or preconceived problems. As we go about our day we could be feeling happy enjoying what the day holds for us. Then some mishap occurs. We get a puncture, we get an unpleasant phone call, maybe something really simple, we spill our coffee. These type of circumstances have the ability to change our mood, sending our thoughts on a downward spiral where negativity seeps in and instead of seeing the mishap or news we received as a blip in an otherwise enjoyable day, we hold on to it and exaggerate it to the point that it can change our feelings and ultimately our mood. Suddenly it's all about this thing in our mind. Instead we could deal with it, acknowledging our feelings surrounding what has happened, then moving on to the next moment and be present with what that holds.

I heard a story about a prisoner of war, who was held captive for about a year. There were thousands of men in the prison camp and in general the conditions were not too bad. The country they were in had a nice climate. The food they were given was fairly good. They had clean water to drink and wash with and a reasonably comfortable place to sleep at night. There was space available to move around inside the compound during the day. No one likes their freedom to be restricted but overall the conditions were fair to good . However there was one exception. Once a day at random, a number of men were chosen and killed by a firing squad. For the on lookers this was harrowing and induced fear everyday as to whether they would be on the list of chosen men. The result was a year of fear, panic, terror and unease caused by the thoughts in their mind of what might be. After a year the camp was closed and the men were free to return to their own country, reunited with their army and families. As time passed and upon reflection the realization was that the year spent there could have been, if not enjoyable, certainly pleasant and easy most of the time. But the thoughts they carried in their minds for the year of what might happen, the possibility of being one of the men chosen for the firing squad, made the year practically unbearable. The constant thought was 'what if it's me tomorrow'? The fear, panic and worry was always in their minds. The terror was in their minds. If they could have spent each day in the present and accepted that they could not alter what might be in the future, the year spent there would have been a totally different experience. Each day lived in the now without thoughts of what might happen the next day is something we have complete control over. No matter what situation we find ourselves in we can decide what thoughts we have and what we allow in our mind.

These of course were quite extreme circumstances. Thankfully we would rarely if ever face something so harrowing. But with any of the stressful or worrisome incidents in our lives, if we accept that we cannot alter the past or future and deal only with the here and now, our lives will be happier.

This is a good story to put things into perspective. How we handle our present moments, and how often when things are going ok or well in our lives, we are the ones who cause unease through our own thoughts? Living and focusing on the present is the route to happiness. It is in ones own mind that this is achievable. Be where you are or you will miss many moments that have the potential for peace and happiness in your life.

Meditation was in the past considered to be the prevail of monks and religious students. Not something that people in general would regularly participate in. Although in recent times it is more commonly practiced. There are lots of techniques, guided meditations and information online to assist in getting us into the habit of using meditation and mindfulness in our daily lives. This is a practice that is accessible to everyone and can be started with only five minutes a day. At home and without any previous experience. Meditation offers positive effects on the mind and body. It is a boost to ones overall wellbeing. To begin, it might feel awkward or difficult but like most things with regular practice, it can become a valuable part of everyday life and will get easier overtime. Finding a comfortable place and relaxing the body and mind. Concentrating on breathing, noticing the intake and exhale of each breath. Focusing solely on breathing. Recognising each thought and letting it go and returning the mind to the present. Breathing and feeling the body. To start with at least, the guided meditation is probably easier as it gives a focus that can assist in helping with wandering thoughts. As we focus on the voice or music guiding us, it offers something to help us concentrate. Inevitably our mind will wonder to begin with. Acknowledge the thought and let it pass. This will stop it leading to another, focusing back to our breathing. Listening and being aware of the feelings within our body. It is difficult to stop the mind wandering but as it becomes part of a daily practice and we slowly increase the minutes we spend at it, so will the time between our mind wandering increase. Once we are in the habit of meditating and practicing mindfulness as we go about our daily business, thoughts that would generally start and mushroom out of control with all manner of negativity, worry and stress, will be caught by our awareness as they arise. The practice of bringing our mind to the present moment will become more frequent and easier.

Sitting alone in a room and being content to enjoy it with no distractions is a difficult task for many people. Alone with the mind can be scary because negative thoughts are much more common than positive ones. Meditation and mindfulness are the tools that if we can get familiar with using, will keep us living in the present. Although we may have difficulties to deal with in the present moment, we always have a choice about the thoughts we allow. Choice is freedom. No matter what we are dealing with we can acknowledge the thought, feel the emotion it evokes, perhaps reframe the thought and then bring the mind back to a state of mindfulness. Even in the moment when being involved with something and without the time to meditate we can press pause. Stop our thoughts, take a deep breath and slowly release it and any stressful feelings.

Mindfulness is purposely giving our focused attention to the present moment and experiencing it without judgment. It is developed by meditation or training. It is a significant part of the Buddhist and Hindu traditions. Mindfulness has been used to reduce depression, stress and anxiety. It has also been used in the treatment of drug addiction, healthy ageing and weight management. There is evidence to suggest that mindfulness meditation may influence physical health and be beneficial to the immune system. It is a source of calming the mind and strengthening the brain.

Yoga is essentially a spiritual practice. It started many centuries ago in ancient India as a meditative practice but is now practiced globally by millions of people. It is a modern choice that offers benefits to the mind and body.

Its aim is to unite the body, mind, soul and universal energy. It includes breathing techniques, relaxation, postures and meditation methods .By ceasing our thoughts we can connect to the source of our being and experience a unity within ourselves. It is a meditation process of self discovery to help see ourselves clearly. To understand and become aware of our thoughts and beliefs .Through practicing yoga we can access resources to help us with self awareness, patience, forgiveness, kindness, love. All positive emotions that are available to us. Practicing yoga, meditation and mindfulness are beneficial for the wellbeing of the mind and body. Although to begin with, setting aside the time in life to incorporate this may seem difficult or even impossible. For most people that do include yoga in their daily schedule, the wellbeing and benefit they experience in time can make these practices a priority in their lives. So introducing them slowly and for a short time is the first step. As the saying goes, 'a thousand mile journey can't happen without the first step'.

The beliefs we hold determine our
success or failure.

We inherit beliefs about ourselves and the
world as we live.

When we are born, we are like a blank canvas. We arrive as a complete perfect being. We don't carry with us a host of beliefs about how things are or should be. But from a young age we are like sponges. Firstly with our parents or care givers then in school with teachers and our peers. We absorb beliefs about ourselves, the world, the people around us and expectations about life. The beliefs that other people in our life or society hold are foisted on us. They enter our conscious and sub conscious mind as we grow and become part of our belief system. These include beliefs about ourselves, our surroundings and form the mindset on how we feel about ourselves. Often these beliefs are self limiting beliefs. They limit our outlook and can be held for the whole of our lives. We can hold these beliefs without questioning them or ever considering why we believe them. Are they true? Is there evidence to support them? Or are these beliefs just something that it's easier to go along with because they have always been part of our lives? Suggested to us and as a result became part of our mindset. A belief can enter our mind simply by a comment someone has made about us. Or a comparison with another person. Growing up, it could be a comparison between siblings. Someone else's opinion that we have taken on and lived by without question. In many cases we don't even remember the origin but it's in our mind and we live by it and behave accordingly.

These beliefs we carry through life can be responsible for our confidence, our self image, our self esteem and feelings about what we expect and deserve in our lives. Living our lives based on beliefs we have picked up from the opinions of others in many cases.

The beliefs we hold about ourselves can be responsible for so many things in our lives. These are a reflection of our thoughts and the voice in our mind. We hear many things everyday. We speak and engage in conversations with many people. But the voice in our head is the one that we listen to most. The constant chatter that goes on as we go about our day. What is that voice telling you? It is important to become aware of it. Is it always putting you down? Suggesting you are not good enough, criticizing what you do, how you look, your capabilities, your worth. Does it negatively compare you to others? Does it berate you for past mistakes? Does it hold grudges from the past? Is it a beneficial or destructive force in your life? Do you ever consider what is true or false in what it tells you? Does it evoke positive or negative feelings when you listen to it?

Do you recognize these types of beliefs?

1 I couldn't join the team, I was never sporty. We're not a sporty family, too weighty for sport. We're big boned. It runs in the family, we've been like this since kids. Sports can be dangerous.

2 I know I've got a temper, got it from my dad. He's the very same. I just lose the head when I get annoyed. It's the way I am. My dad and me have always been like that. Can't help it. Born like that. Can't change who you are.

3 I got a wedding invitation for myself and a friend. Don't know who I can invite. I'd love to ask Mary. She's lovely but she would never go with me. We get on well, chatting in work but she's so pretty. She'd never come out with me. Bet she thinks I'm overweight and not good looking. She probably chats to me because she feels sorry for me. She's really clever too and good at her job. Probably thinks I'm stupid. I can't ask her to come with me.

These examples are the type of beliefs that people form in their minds but are not based on facts. They believe them because of suggestions or ideas they have picked up. It's easier to accept them than to question them. In some cases without even an awareness of these beliefs or how they are holding us back in life, they add negativity to life and can become more ingrained over a lifetime and accepted as reality. When in fact they are really just beliefs not based on fact. They are self limiting beliefs. I've heard them described as internal tattoos and I think that's a good description for understanding them. Like an addition to our minds .

Referred to as self limiting beliefs because they limit how we feel about ourselves and the life we are living, often not true, they are perfect fodder for negative internal mind chatter. They give reason for not trying or accomplishing things in life which could be enjoyable and /or benifital. They can be responsible for negative comparisons wo make about ourselves.

A useful exercise to become aware of how we feel about ourselves and what we tell ourselves, is to write a description of our self. Being as honest as we can and write what we believe to be our values, interests, what we like and dislike. What are our strengths and weaknesses? Are the things we believe about our self true? Are they others observations or suggestions? Do we see ourselves in a positive or negative light? Are we happy with the description? Are there things we would like to change? We can make changes in our mind. That is the first step to changing anything in our life. Believe it to be true.

Imposter syndrome is when people doubt their own skills, talents and what they have accomplished in life. It is self doubt and the feeling of incompetence. It is a belief that they do not deserve the success or the reward for their achievements. They put their accomplishments down to luck or circumstances and worry that they will be regarded as a fraud and lose creditability. They are fearful that they won't live up to the expectation of others and often, the more they achieve the more they doubt themselves.

These type of feelings can induce negative self talk and feelings of failure. They can cause one to put excessive pressure on themselves. They find it hard to accept that everyone makes mistakes and they feel the need to be a perfectionist. This can be common when trying new things, which in turn can prevent them from pursuing goals and taking up opportunities as they arise. Comparisons to other people and their achievements can give them a feeling of inferiority. Social media is one area that can give rise to those feelings as it can portray people to be leading the perfect life. If one believes everything that is seen there, it can lead to an inferior sense of self.

Measuring our own achievements without comparison to others. Listing our accomplishments and knowing that at times when we make a mistake, it is an opportunity to learn. Also, talking these type of feelings over with a trusted friend can help to have them acknowledge that our achievements are well deserved.

When we become aware of the voice in our head, we will not only realise that past and future events and scenarios are constantly being brought into the present moment of our lives. But also that comparisons are being made with other people. When we constantly hear negative chatter about ourselves it reinforces what the belief is and we can live and act in accordance to those beliefs, which are nothing more than suggestions or accusations about ourselves that have become ingrained in our mindset. As we go through life we all make mistakes and our hope is to learn from them. Unfortunately from a young age our mistakes can be looked upon as who we are. We are not the mistakes we make or made. If we do not excel academically, we could be labelled as stupid but we might be a genius with practical tasks. We may be slow on a sport pitch and labelled lazy but excel at art and be energetic when involved in that. So it's important not to label people based on how they preform at particular tasks. This unfortunately can be common practice in our formative years.

It is difficult to go through life without comparisons to other people. From an early age we are compared in our developmental stages. In school we are rated as to our results in class. Socially there are suggested mile stones as we approach adult life. This continues for most if not all of our lives. There are social norms like getting what is perceived to be a good job, a life partner, a property, having a family. There is of course nothing wrong with having any of these things in life. But we are not all the same and as Albert Einstein said, 'If you judged all creatures in completing a task to climb a tree, obviously the monkey will excel far better than the fish.' Comparisons with people are just as unrealistic. Comparisons that people make can give rise to thoughts of failure or of not being as successful or as smart as others these comparisons limit the person and can lead to thoughts of lack and failure. Our thoughts lead to feelings. Feelings that result from these type of negative thoughts are feelings that do not serve us well and are often the result of false beliefs.

I have spoken recently to a few late 20s to 30 year olds who have spent the years from leaving school either travelling or going from job to job. They often describe a sense of panic caused by a belief that their life is going by and they should have achieved something stable and be 'set up 'with what is perceived as 'a successful' life . These feelings can rob them of the enjoyment of their day to day lives. Rather they could consider every day a success with whatever they are choosing to do each day. Planning and having goals is positive but not if we miss the day we've been given by thoughts of panic about our future. Or if we experience feelings of failure because we haven't reached some perceived socially accepted norm by a certain age, then life itself can be missed. We have all been given a certain amount of days to live and none of us know how many. So each day no matter how far through the journey we are, the day you are in is the most important one. Don't lose out on that one worrying about future ones that are not guaranteed. There can be thoughts of 'I tried this or that' and it didn't work out, so I wasted time on it. We don't waste our time if we are present while we are involved with what we are doing. We may not always get the result we want. But we have experienced the time and have had the opportunity to learn from it.

Some people who are considered to be most successful in their lives didn't gain that success until later in life. Just like the comparisons to people's abilities, comparisons as to the age at which people are perceived to reach certain goals is just as unrealistic. We are all on our own journey. Our lives unfold when the time is right for each individual. We shouldn't put ourselves under pressure to a perceived time line.

We hear about extreme cases where a child has been abused or neglected physically or verbally during their childhood and mental health problems often ensue in their adult life as a result of this abusive childhood. There is an excepted connection.

But for most people where there isn't anything extreme about the childhood there is still a constant flow of suggestions, accusations, expectations and comparisons. Not just as we grow up but constantly throughout our whole life. We are constantly fed information more so than ever before, with technology and media becoming more and more a part of our daily life. They offer constant suggestions about how we should be living. What a successful life looks like. What the perfect image is. How we should aspire to live our lives to conform to this suggested role of perfection.

If we can somehow manage to conform and achieve all the suggestions, then we will have the perfect life and be happy. But the majority of these suggestions for a happy life are things that come from outside sources. However it is only possible to find happiness from within oneself. So what is this constant information we are taking in on a daily basis? In a lot of cases it is making people feel inferior because after striving to build what is suggested as the perfect life when fulfilment and happiness are not achieved, it gives a feeling of failure as we continue to strive for happiness from outside sources. Looking within is the only place to obtain happiness. The limits in our life are created by our mind.

Happiness is often confused with pleasure. We can all gain pleasure from things in life. Pleasurable things add to our life's enjoyment and are not a problem in most cases. But taking pleasure from something is different than using or obtaining it to bring happiness into your life. To understand and define the difference, pleasure comes from outside sources, things outside of ourselves which we enjoy. But to gain true happiness it is only attainable from within.

I read a short story recently about two people who went in search of a new location to live. The first one arrived at a village he was considering a move to. He had a walk around and came upon a local man. He stopped to have a chat and find out some things about the village. He asked the local man 'what type of village is this, is it a friendly place, is there a friendly community'? The local man replied with a question, 'tell me' he said, 'what was the village like that you have come from, how did you find it there'? The visitor answered, 'it was a very nice place, the people were friendly and there was a great community spirit'. 'Ah well' said the local, 'you will find the same thing here'! Further along the road the local man met the other visitor who was considering a move there. He stopped to talk again, this visitor asked the same question about the village and the people there, were they friendly and welcoming. The local man answered with the same question, "how did you like the last place you lived"? The visitor answered, 'I didn't like the people there, not friendly or welcoming, a miserable place really.' 'Ah well' said the local, 'I'm sure you will find the same here'!

The local was basically saying to both men, what you bring with you, how you feel and interact with the people you meet is the reality you will experience.

What is inside us is what we project out to the people around us. If we are happy and satisfied with our lives, living and enjoying the moment as it is happening, that is what comes across to other people and that is what they respond to. They get a feeling of happiness from us, a positive vibe which is coming across. This makes it likely that they will respond positively to us. Of course in life we can be happy and fulfilled and meet someone who is living a totally different reality and is so entrenched in their own negative thoughts that the positive outlook you exude cannot even penetrate their thoughts. One of the signs as to whether someone is enjoying a happy life is if they are taking responsibility for the choices and experiences in their life. People who constantly blame external factors or other people for how their lives are unfolding are normally unhappy. They hold everyone from the government to their family to their employers responsible for their feelings. Focusing constantly on outer sources and not looking within themselves. It is easy if we look outside ourselves to find endless problems and people to blame. Unfortunately there are many people that live their lives with a mindset of, 'it's not my fault, I can't change it.' 'Someone else must fix it for me, it's not fair.' This attitude is giving our power away. Blaming external factors for our problems can hinder our resilience and skills at coping with life's challenges.

We need to be able to deal with life's ups and downs. Otherwise we live with feelings of being helpless. To enjoy life we each need to take responsibility for the life we are living.

If we are living in awareness of how our thoughts affect our happiness, we won't feel the need to take on other people's unhappiness. We can send them love, perhaps silently and move on, knowing that their happiness can only be obtained from within themselves. The awareness of their thoughts, leads to their feelings and to a mindset of happiness.

Our thoughts are the basis of a happy life. Our lives are a collection of now moments. If we are having positive, pleasant, grateful thoughts, the collection of these in the now moment is what gives us the experience of a happy life. People spend their lives focusing on so many things outside themselves, looking for the success they feel will bring them happiness. But really the best success IS happiness. By focusing on the now moments in our lives the success of happiness is possible. Isn't it a good feeling to realise that "now" is the only moment we have to deal with? We always only have to deal with now. When we realise and accept that, everything becomes clear. It is our mind and our thoughts that bring the feelings that we don't want or like into our life.

Noticing what makes us feel good. When we are feeling good, Considering what it is that we are experiencing. If we can identify people and situations that give us a good feeling, it's like bottling it! We can return to it.

Also doing the same with situations and people that bring feelings of negativity to us. When we identify these, we can choose not to engage with them. Or in some cases with family or work perhaps, we can't do that. But by being aware of it, we can decide the thoughts we bring to each situation and can decide to respond rather than react. This makes it easier to navigate our way around the situation.

Our minds and thoughts are central to our feelings. Like any other part of the body they need to be nourished. When we speaks of nourishment for the body, we immediately consider the food we eat. (This is also a vital part of maintaining a healthy mind and body). We can for the most part recognise foods that are healthy and nourishing as opposed to food that is unhealthy or gone off. We wouldn't eat something that we thought would make us feel ill. We need to be as aware of what we feed our minds. Is what we watch, read and listen to from the media, in print or TV and radio nourishing our minds? Or are we consuming a daily dose of fear and negativity? The people we spend our time with, are they positive, loving, caring, helpful people. Or are they complaining, angry, stressed, argumentative people? What goes into our minds will effect our thoughts. There are so many beautiful things that we can nourish our minds with daily but we must make it a habit to seek them out and appreciate them.

Have you noticed when advertisers are using before and after photos to sell products, the before photo doesn't have a smiling face? But the after one does! Because a smile alone can transform the face. The muscles we use to smile lift the face and gives a more attractive and youthful look. Smiling can also reduce stress, improve how we feel and helps us feel happy because it makes us feel more relaxed. If we don't feel like smiling but consciously do it anyway it will still have a positive effect on how we feel. A smile makes us more approachable to others. It gives us a look of confidence, competence and being relaxed. It is a sign that everyone recognises. It changes the whole face and brightens the eyes. It has the ability to say 'welcome' without verbal communication. A smile can change our mood and that of the people we interact with. We can't always know as we go about our day what difficulty the people we come into contact with are experiencing. Something as simple as smiling at others has the power to add positive change to their day and ours. A smile can be contagious! As we smile at others they involuntary smile back in most cases. A smile can be described as a natural boost to our overall health and well being. Like an inbuilt mood changer! We spend a lot of cash on products to make ourselves look better but wearing a smile is probably the cheapest and one of the most effective ways to look and feel good.

Recently I visited a friend who has experienced a botrayal by someone very close in her life and is working through healing from it. We were having a conversation about it and strange as it may seem, we started to put a humorous perspective on the whole incident which gained momentum and suddenly the two of us were in fits of laughter. Like really contagious belly laughter! In fact at one point, she stood up and was bent over trying to stop laughing! We both felt so much better after this. It didn't change what had happened but having a good laugh can be so beneficial. It brings focus away from the anger, guilt, stress, whatever negativity is being experienced but it has much more benefits than just being a distraction.

Laughter induces many physical changes in the body. A bout of laughter increases oxygen intake and stimulates the bodies organs. Our heart, lungs and circulation. It also helps to relax muscles. The immune system can be strengthened by laughter. It is overall beneficial to our well being. It is something that can help when dealing with difficult situations and helps to connect people, as it is an emotion that is contagious. A good laugh can be shared in company, we could all use more laughter in life. Children laugh much more than adults so it is obviously something that we do less of as we grow. But it is worth being conscious of and seeking ways to have a good laugh and experience the many positive rewards.

Figuring out what makes us feel good and making a habit to include it in our lives is so beneficial. Dancing is a big mood changer for me. It doesn't have to be on a night out, although I do love that. Having upbeat, happy music play as I'm cooking or cleaning, particularly washing windows or floors and bopping along to the music, makes the tasks more enjoyable. Plus I get the benefit of the exercise! It may not be dancing in the kitchen for you. Although if you haven't tried it, I do recommend it! But whatever lifts you and is a mood changer, make it a habit in your life.

As we go about our daily lives, one of the beliefs that seems to be commonly held is that we should constantly be on the go, being productive, achieving something each day to further us along our life path. To constantly strive to get things done is often the main focus in life. There seems to be a sense of guilt attached to spending time doing nothing. But time perceived as wasted, can actually be time spent choosing to rest, looking after ourselves, nourishing our minds, switching off from the outside world, listening to our bodies and mind and being silent. We should in fact feel a sense of achievement at giving ourselves the gift of being. Unfortunately doing nothing or being lazy as it can be referred to has negative connotations. It can cause feelings of guilt but as humans time to rest and relax are valid necessities to keep our mind and bodies healthy. So allowing yourself time to just BE is really important. Perhaps try the experience of taking a few hours away from your normal life. Leave your phone or anything else which could disturb you. Find a quiet place alone. Absorb the silence and just BE. Be in the moment and enjoy the gift of that present time. Whether we are resting or taking time out, it is the awareness of keeping our minds focused on the present and the time we have to enjoy that is what will keep our minds free from negativity.

The limiting beliefs we hold about ourselves can be a large part of the thoughts that go on in our minds. Without even realising it we constantly say things like, oh I'm too old or I'm too fat. I couldn't do that I'm not clever enough or I'm not pretty enough. Apart from believing these thoughts, we actually reinforce this negativity in our mind. This is destructive behavior. I'm sure it's easy to accept that if we were to tell a child that they were stupid every day, they would grow up believing it. But even as adults we tell ourselves negative things constantly in our minds. We often do it subconsciously but awareness of what we are saying to ourselves is the first step to change. A good exercise is to write a list of all the positives about ourselves. Starting each comment with I Am. This is affirming how we feel about ourselves and enters our subconscious. The more we can affirm to ourselves the positive things we believe about ourselves, the more they will become apart of our mind and subconscious mind. We will begin to feel what we tell ourselves over time. I am happy, I am healthy, I am loved, I am smart, etc. If we find ourselves talking negatively about ourselves, we must change that thought and consider something positive we feel about ourselves and replace the thought with that. Reframe the negative to a positive thought. E.g. I'm too old -to- I have many years of life experience. Or I couldn't do that -to- I have the opportunity to try something new.

Another commonly held belief is to live thinking that when I get my new house, new job, lose weight, meet a partner whatever it is we desire, things will be well and I will be happy. Looking to the future with a plan of what we want and having goals and working towards achieving them is good. But happiness won't be achieved that way because when your desire comes to pass, you will no doubt desire something else and your life will be lived focusing on the future and what you want to obtain, somehow imagining that that's the thing that will bring happiness. It is inside yourself that happiness is achieved. Your desires can still be achieved but are not the route to happiness.

Living in the past or looking back with dissatisfaction can keep us stuck from new beginnings and a fulfilling life. It's more common now for people to go through life and experience more than one long term relationship or marriage. Because this is something that has changed in the last few generations, there is for some people an association of failure in relationship breakdown. It is often a difficult time and a big change when we are coping with a breakdown of a relationship and for some people it's extremely hard to move on. Perhaps because they feel they can't cope without their ex partner or that life will never be as good. Or they apply blame which leads to bitterness about why or how the relationship ended. I know people who have been apart for many years and have not moved on. They still see their situation as a failure on theirs or usually on their ex's part. They blame everything that has happened since on the fact that they are not with their partner any more. They don't consider meeting someone new. They are closed from the possibility of that by the hurt and blame they carry with them from the past relationship. They never reach a point of being happy with their single status. To be happy in a relationship I think one needs to be happy being alone. No other person can or should be responsible for your happiness, it has to be an inside job. People secure in their own lives and responsible for themselves are the most likely to have a successful relationship with another. I've had 3 long term relationships. Two were marriages and at some point in each one it was time for it to end and for us both to move on separately. At the time it's not always easy and there is a period of adjusting. But to hold on to hurt and blame for the other person is just hurting yourself. I've heard it described as 'drinking poison and expecting the other person to die'!

Any blame for someone else we carry with us from the past, has the affect of hurting us and being destructive to our present and future. It can take time to heal ourselves from a broken relationship but the best thing we can do for ourselves is to forgive the other person any blame we attribute to them and move on without reliving the incidents that we feel wronged by. Accept that it is over. It was a period of our life and it's possible that the next period can offer us something better if we can be open to it. There was obviously a time when we wanted to be with the person and probably a period that was good. It is better to think of the time we were happily together as a success and it was a success that when the time came, the right thing to do was to move on. That is not a failure that is a success if we move on and start living life again and decide on the future we want. Some relationships and marriages last, 'until death do us part,' and in cases that the couples are happy together, that's fantastic and probably what most people who enter a relationship hope for. But it's not like that for everyone, but that doesn't mean it's a failure or one should live on in regret. For some people forgiving the other person, appears to be accepting the wrongs they consider were done to them and condoning the actions of the other person. But as we know we are not in control of the actions of others and not responsible for them. By forgiving we are doing this for ourselves, we are in control of our own feeling and taking responsibility for ourselves. When we feel hurt by someone, it's not unusual to want the last word on the subject, or consider taking revenge. But this just keeps the hurt going as part of our life as we relive it over and over in our mind. Not engaging or reacting is probably the most helpful response. At least until we can get to a place of forgiveness or indifference to the person. Then genuinely release the person with no negativity and move on. Of course it's not only romantic relationships that come and go in our lives. Friends can let us down or hurt us and we move on. But it's the moving on and forgiving without blame that is the success part. There are often triggers that bring up past or unpleasant thoughts and feelings. It is a worthwhile exercise to become conscious of these. Some might be obvious and easy to identify. Others more subtle but whether it is a person a place or a type of situation, bringing awareness of it to our thoughts and either avoiding it if possible or deciding to respond rather that react, will take the power out of whatever it is that triggers negativity for us. Writing or journaling which is becoming more common these days, is a great way to look at what is happening. Or when questions come into our mind, we can find a sense of release by putting things on paper. It nearly feels like we can take it from the mind and give it to the paper! We can stimulate answers to questions as we write them, like working towards a solution by taking the time and thought to write it. This can be very helpful with unpleasant situations from our past which we are trying to clear from our mind. Writing and destroying the paper is like an unloading from the mind and a permanent release of it. It is a physical action to rid the mind from something. Anything negative from the past that we continue to carry with us is like wearing a heavy backpack as we go about our day. Just consider how much relief is experienced by taking off a heavy backpack and moving on. Releasing old hurts, regrets, disappointments from our past gives similar relief.

How we get along with other people in our lives and how we treat them has a direct impact on our own life. When we converse with others our ability to listen is an important factor. In many cases we can be very intent on answering and thinking of the next thing we want to say ourselves. Perceived conversation can get in the way of real dialogue. Really listening requires being present. We need to discover listening with all of our senses. To really know what is being said, the body language, facial expressions and the emotions of the other person can all tell as much as the spoken word. This is the experience of real engagement with another in the present moment.

Expect the best. That is what we deserve.

Deciding how our reality will be and
create that reality.

We can't of course stop our minds thinking nor would we want to. Everything comes from a thought or idea before it becomes a reality. We create with our minds. There is a vast difference between the internal chatter that is destructive in our minds and the intentional focused thinking and creating that is possible. The law of attraction is the universal law that states that what we focus on, we attract into our lives. Whatever we give our energy and attention to will enter our life. As in, like attracts like but to a degree, what we expect is what becomes reality. It is the feelings and expectations of thoughts that bring about what comes into our lives. If we focus on and concern ourselves with negative future events we create the feelings associated with negativity and can bring about these negative events. Because our minds react to suggestion even when we do not often realise it.

I experienced this when I was giving birth to my son. I had gone to the hospital because my waters had broken. I was not experiencing any pain. I was made comfortable in a bed. A nurse said that a midwife would be along shortly to examine me. It was all very calm. My partner was with me and I had no pain. I thought I had a long time to wait before anything would start happening. The midwife arrived and examined me and with surprise in her voice declared that this is not going to take long. 'You are nearly fully dilated'. The moment I heard those words I began to experience pain! Immediately! That continued until my beautiful son was delivered. This was a very strong indication to me of how suggestive the mind is. I thought I had not even really started labour and as such my mind was reacting to that reality. I was calm and not experiencing any pain. But when I was told that in fact I WAS in labour and at the late stages, my mind and body reacted to what is expected at that stage which is severe pain and that is what I experienced.

This experience made me realise how strong the power of

suggestion is and what we expect is what we experience in our reality. There is the saying about the glass half empty or half full. Some people expect life to work out as they want. Perhaps it comes down to self esteem and what they feel they deserve. For some they have come to figure out from books and teachings, the connection between our expectations and our reality. The realisation has sparked the awareness and then consciously an effort is made to expect the best. But it obviously works both ways and for people who have expectations of difficulty, lack, illness and hardship their expectations are as likely to create THAT reality. It can have a continuing effect both ways. If we expect good things and that is what we get then we are more likely to feel great. Things are going well and we keep our expectations high. Living from a place of positive expectation produces a positive reality. But from the outlook of expecting the worst and getting it, we then consider thoughts like, things never work out for me, and it keeps us on the receiving end of a difficult reality.

I worked with a girl some years ago. She was a single parent and seemed to concentrate a lot on the fact that if she got sick and couldn't work it would be a disastrous situation. With two children to rear and a mortgage, she often looked at insurance plans for illness and remortgage options in the event that some illness might befall her. She brought the subject up on many occasions. At the time I did feel it was a real concern that she lived with. Years later with her children reared and out doing well and making their own way in the world, she did in fact get seriously ill. By that time she had married and didn't have to deal with the situation alone. Although it took her a long time to be back on her feet, thankfully she made a full recovery. None of the concerns she feared about getting ill were relevant when the illness occurred. Had she attracted the illness into her life with the attention she had given it for years? Had she given her body the expectation that it was coming?

The law of attraction suggests that the good and the bad that we focus our attention on can enter our lives. We are the creators of our reality by the thoughts we nurture and where we put our focused attention. With awareness, we can focus and create expectations for the things we want in our reality.

There is a very real correlation between how our outlook, our thoughts and expectation affect our lives. If we constantly believe and reinforce limiting beliefs about ourselves and our lives, speaking them in our mind, we are by our own words and thoughts bringing about our reality.

Without an awareness of how powerful suggestion and expectation in, we can create all manner of negativity in our lives. Considering again the things that are suggested to us, from conversations we have to the media, all these things are absorbed regularly into our thoughts and create feelings in our day to day lives.

When we are mindful of how we phrase our thoughts and words, we begin to notice when speaking with others how common it is for people to talk negatively about a situation. Eg. I'm no good at interviews ,I probably won't get the job or my flights are always delayed when I go on holiday. I doubt my car will pass the test. We need to reframe those thoughts to, I have the ability to do a good interview and am looking forward to being offered the job. I look forward to easy, stress-free travel to my holiday. I'm pleased that my car will be tested and pass.

In the media it is frequently reported that the cost of living is going out of control. Working people are finding themselves homeless. There are possibly more health epidemics on the way. The planet is likely to burn up with global warming. When these disasters are reported world wide and the collective conscious reacts to the suggestion of these events, it is like a global expectation of negativity. We react to what is being suggested and the feelings they induce in us collectively are real. All brought about by suggestion. In many cases the events will not directly affect the listeners' life and not at that moment but it is being taken into the global subconscious.

Most of the worlds' population were effected in 2020 by the COVID pandemic. But to varying degrees. Some people lost loved ones which of course was sad and difficult. Some people felt they lost a year or more of their life. Some lived for the complete duration in a state of fear and panic in case they would succumb to the virus. It's a bit like the story of the war prisoners earlier In the book. On a daily basis for the people that weren't sick which was the majority of the population, it was all down to how you reacted to it. How we received it and framed our thoughts around it. Unfortunately it has been reported that many suffered with mental health problems as a result of it. I feel blessed to have enjoyed it. I focused on all the positives and I really felt they WERE positives. I had time (although mainly at home) to do as I pleased. I cooked, read, sewed and crocheted. I did jigsaws and enjoyed many long and interesting conversations with friends on the phone. I'd wake each morning and start the day with an online group studying a chapter of the book, The Magic by Rhonda Byrne. Then I would decide how I would spend my day on something I enjoyed.

I spent so much time doing things that ordinarily would be considered leisure activities and a waste of time and possible source of feelings of guilt. However at that time it was considered a great achievement to be occupying the day and living happily! Partly through this period I realised that anything I enjoy doing is never a waste of time or something to feel any guilt about. I accepted that my life is meant to be about enjoyment and spending my time how I wish. Guilt is a destructive emotion that serves no purpose. Slowing down also makes us aware of how our life is. When we are constantly on the go and moving too fast we can miss what's happening but with a period of slowing down, it can help us to make clearer choices and cause us to respond rather than to react and appreciate just BEING.

Had we been given notice, maybe a month with the expectation of being house bound and restricted for weeks, I would not have imagined that it could be an enjoyable experience. But as it unfolded without knowing how long it would continue, it could be dealt with on a day to day basis. I was, for the duration of the pandemic in Spain and living alone. The lockdown lasted for about 10 weeks and was very heavily policed as regards how far we could travel from our house and for what reason. I know in some places it wasn't as strict and more movement outside was possible. But if we accept that we have choice in any situation because of our thoughts, our thoughts offer freedom. How we frame what is happening is what makes the difference.

We can with awareness be conscious of the suggestions that we let into our thoughts. We can decide how we want our lives to look and work for us and WE can create the suggestions. There is plenty of beauty in this world. Beautiful people, beautiful places, beauty in nature, enjoyable things to do. We can focus on these things and show gratitude for the beauty that surrounds us and the ability to take part in things we enjoy.

Can you imagine if all the media and news agencies decided for a day that everything that was transmitted for a 24hr period was going to look at some positive event, or beautiful happening? All the goodness in the world was celebrated in this 24 hr period. Some people may think there probably isn't enough good things happening in the world to report on for 24 hrs. But there is plenty of positivity. It is just that bad news sells better. Negative events are the common fodder of the media. To decide to give up listening to news or reading news paper or news reels on social media is an act of removing a vast amount of negativity from our everyday lives. But if it changed for a period and the outlook relayed was positive, upbeat, wholesome and happy. As a global collective consciousness, isn't it possible that the feelings and reactions would be different? Our reaction to this beauty and positivity could change our mindset and on a global scale we might experience a brighter reality.

Affirmations can change our mindset. An Affirmation is a spoken or written sentence affirming a belief we accept. It's our choice whether we affirm positive thoughts or negative ones about ourselves and the world around us. Considering what the beliefs we carry around in our thoughts and reframe the negatives to positives and getting into the habit of affirming the new beliefs to ourselves regularly can change our mindset.

E.g. I believe in my abilities and can achieve what I desire

I have no worries and I focus on what I can control

I am proud of myself and my achievements

All is perfectly well in my world. (This is a favorite of mine)

These are just examples. Affirmations can relate to anything in our life. Anything about ourselves or the world that we doubt or worry about can be reframed in an affirmation and read or spoken aloud to change the mindset we hold and to suggest to ourselves and affirm a new thought and belief. Earlier I spoke of worry and how my mother worried. It is very common for people to use these words in relation to themselves or others ,"I'm really worried about" followed by what is on their mind. If we change that to an affirmation, it is so much more powerful and positive. So instead of putting out the verbal negative affirmations of I'm so worried ,my friend is unwell reframe it and affirm my friend is well and visually see her completely recovered. There is no incident or time when worry is of any value. Although for some people it's difficult to stop worrying thoughts. However with an awareness of how futile it is, accepting that an affirmation about the situation offers so much more positive energy to it can be a way to change our mindset. When we feel a thought of "I'm worried" getting into the habit of reframing it to a positive affirmation will make a difference. What we say when we use the word worry is a negative affirmation.

Our thoughts, words, expectations, feelings and suggestions, are all responsible for our experiences and the reality in our lives.

The law of attraction states that we can attract into our lives what we desire and usually the focus on videos etc. with regard to this, is on six figure salaries and luxuries such as mansions and yachts. These are outer pleasures which many people want to obtain. But inner happiness is very much obtainable by thoughts, expectations, feelings and suggestions. If we can obtain inner happiness, the worldly luxuries will not be our main focus because it is more beneficial to be grateful for what we have got, rather than looking outside ourselves for pleasure from worldly goods.

I am not suggesting that to be happy we cannot live in luxury with everything that money can buy. Of course we can, but worldly luxuries and pleasurable items alone will not bring us happiness. We can live happy and fulfilling lives with few material luxuries because real happiness is gained from within ourselves.

Living a life of positive expectation is a good way I think to describe the law of attraction. If you had a wish for a particular thing to happen in your life and it came to pass, or you somehow knew that what you wanted was imminent, apart from the feeling of expectation, there are the feelings you get once the desire has presented itself. Feelings of achievement, feelings of gratitude and excitement perhaps and plans to be put in place to facilitate it. When we have an expectation and we really believe it will happen, those feelings can come before the arrival and add to the overall expectation. Focusing on our desires and what we want to receive or accomplish is the start to creating them, then taking action that could assist in the existence of the desire.

Vision boards are a popular way of putting the experiences and desires you want to attract into your life in your sight everyday. It can be fun and enjoyable to create a vision board. Creating a board with pictures or affirmations of what you want to attract into your life is a wonderful exercise. The visual impact of regularly seeing these things puts them into your conscious and subconscious mind regularly. The law of attraction states that what we focus our mind on, we attract into our reality .

Often to realise what we do want, we come from thoughts of what we don't want. This is putting negative feeling and energy towards our desires and how we frame what we are trying to attract. It is important to word and feel the desire from a positive aspect .

But to put constant focus on the fact that the desire has not yet materialised puts the wrong focus upon it. That is putting the focus on lack and creating a feeling of lack. If it is something that is to come into your life and the energy you surround the thoughts with are positive, you can then expect that it will come without chasing or panic. Rather with flow and expectation, believing and allowing things to unfold in the perfect timing for you.

Think of it like this. A townland is suffering the devastating effects of drought The people come together to pray for rain, to do a rain dance, anything that they feel can make the rain come. About 100 People show up, to try to bring some rain. But only one young boy brings an umbrella. That is true expectation.

The start of our day is an ideal time to give consideration to the awareness of our thoughts. When we awake and our day is before us, we know the things we are planning to spend our time on doing that day. Sometimes of course the day will have things that we are excited about doing. Other days will feel like a day of chores lies ahead or things we just need to get through, which we don't hold much enthusiasm for. When the day ahead doesn't seem to hold much to look forward to, it's easy to start with thoughts of, "I really don't want to go here or to do that". Then we can let our minds wander to what could go wrong, to the stresses and hassles that could be involved. We chatter along in our minds about all the things we don't want to do but must do during the day. Which results in us starting our day with the expectation of a miserable one, dragging ourselves out of bed with a feeling of dread.

Instead, consciously picturing the perfect day. Seeing everything that we are doing working out perfectly, being easy to accomplish and enjoyable. As we start to ready ourselves for the day using affirmations to affirm the good day ahead.

Eg. I will accomplish with ease and enjoyment the things I do today.

I am grateful for this perfect day where all things work out for my good.

These type of affirmations to begin the day will give us a mindset of a good day ahead. Apart from just saying them expecting what we are saying to be completely true. Whatever we are going to do that day, imagining the enjoyment of doing it and its perfect completion. Deciding on having a good day and expecting it . Our mindset at the beginning of the day will have an affect on how the day unfolds.

A few years ago, I was contacted by a local solicitor. He had been to the local court that day and heard my name being called in relation to a traffic offence. I had been away and had not received any notification about it. So with my failure to appear in court, a warrant had been issued for my arrest! He advised me of the next court case and told me I really must attend. I was initially shocked at hearing about a warrant being issued. I put it from my mind until the morning I had to go to court. Then I focused my mind on my leaving the court. I knew there was a ladies boutique opposite the court and I saw myself walking out the door of the court with a smile on my face, crossing the road and looking in the boutique window. This was a vivid picture with details that I had in my mind and the complete expectation that it would happen like that. I was smiling and I had a good feeling in my focused visualisation. I went to court and the situation was dealt with in minutes. I left the court without a fine or any repercussion and then in reality I did walk across the road smiling and looked in the window of the boutique feeling good.

This is the type of scenario that could have had me

stressed for the couple of weeks as I waited for the day in question. I could have spent so much time imagining the worst. A huge fine! How would I pay it? Might I lose my driving license? etc. But I didn't let any of those thoughts enter my mind. I only let the thoughts of the outcome I wanted run through my mind. I expected that I would get the outcome I wanted. I accept that I was focusing on an event that was in the future but it was with awareness of the positive outcome I wanted and it was inducing the feelings of happiness and gratitude I would feel while leaving the court. This is entirely different to letting our mind wander to possible outcomes taking place that we don't want and can cause feelings of panic or stress. This was a positive visualisation with the feelings and expectation that the situation would untold as I decided .

Becoming aware of our minds and what we are thinking and feeling, what we are expecting in our life can be put in place for incidents such as I dealt with on that day. However we can do it on a daily basis when it's a routine day for us. We can put in place the expectation of a good day, a day we feel good and everything works out well in our world.

There are common factors in all our lives that if we can get to work positively for us, can be the essence of living a contended and happy life.

Health, relationships, finances, community, friends, career, diet, sleep, spiritual beliefs, hobbies, outlook, goals, change.

All of these areas of life can be improved by affirming verbally we want them to be and believing it, which can in turn change our mindset around them.

Here is an Affirmation for each one or you can write your own in the page set out in the back of the book.

Health

I enjoy perfect health. My body and mind are healthy and happy and are a blessing which I am grateful to enjoy.

Relationships

My relationship is loving, caring, honest and fun. We are both in a perfect place and are nourished by each other.

Wealth

Wealth flows constantly and easily into my life. I am open to all the abundance that I receive.

Community

I am one part of the larger community. We each have something to offer and I am grateful for what I give and receive.

Friends

My friendships are important to me, and I will nurture and cherish them. I can rely on my friends and trust them to be there for me.

Career

I am grateful to have a career. My skills are valuable and appreciated. I give to my work and am rewarded.

Diet

I enjoy healthy nourishing food daily which is satisfying to eat and fuels my mind and body. It keeps me healthy. Thank you for the blessing of eating well each day.

Sleep

I have a comfortable, warm peaceful place to sleep at night. I sleep well and am revitalised for a new day. The sleep I get is a perfect refresher for the day ahead.

Spiritual beliefs.

I am part of source energy. To trust this connection is all I need to live without fear. All creation is worthy of this.

Hobbies

I have time and energy and creative talent to enjoy my hobbies. Enjoyment of my hobbies is an asset to my mindset and reality.

Outlook

My outlook is positive. I feel and exude positive energy. I am open to all the positive opportunity and interaction which I experience in my life.

Goals

I am ready, willing and able to achieve my goals. I am confident in my ability and know I will succeed.

Change

My life is unfolding in perfect timing to a perfect plan. I am living with a belief that my life will flow easily and any changes I don't foresee are for my good.

When we read these we might think, well I don't have all that. But that is the way to receive it. Believe that we are worthy of what we want and constantly affirm it in our mind. Being sure to word our affirmations from a positive viewpoint. Eg. "I am happy and healthy" as opposed to " I don't want to be sick and depressed any longer". It makes a difference with thoughts and words, when talking about ourselves or situations, to do so coming from a positive perspective.

Gratitude is one of the ways to change our thoughts and feelings. Unfortunately some people feel they have little to be grateful for and concentrate on what they feel is missing in their lives. Because their wish list of the things they feel are missing in their lives is long they have a mindset of lack, always wishing and wanting for more. But for anyone living there are things to be grateful for. We can start with all the things that are commonly taken for granted. Actively looking for things to be grateful for. Such as the beauty of nature that surrounds us, the air we breathe, the day we have been given, the people we know. The list can be endless and different for everyone. Bringing feelings of gratitude into our livoe can change our mindset to one of optimism thus improving our day to day life. Being grateful can positively improve many areas of our life by increasing happiness and feeling better about ourselves. It helps interaction with others and our overall well being both when we are going about our day or during our sleep. All are influenced by experiencing gratitude. We can give gratitude for things we desire to enter our lives. Even if we are experiencing an illness, to give gratitude for our perfect health is suggesting to our mind that is our current state. It is common when people feel under the weather, to constantly tell themselves and others how bad they are feeling. This induces further feelings of ill health. Being grateful for abundance even when we feel areas of our lives are lacking is to give positive affirmation to the mind and so induce better feelings. The habit of gratitude can change our feelings and with that the reality we experience.

In what appears to be a difficult or sad situation, if we

are willing to change the way we look at it, we will find something to be grateful for. One of the most difficult events we experience in our lives can be the loss of a loved one and feeling of loss, sadness, anger are all appropriate emotions to experience in this situation. It is natural to go through a grieving period. But we can also be grateful for the wonderful gift of having had this person in our life for the time that we did. Grateful for what they added to our life, for the time, experiences, love and all the wonderful things about them that are the reason we miss them.

As with other difficulties we face, from life changing ones to minor ones, how we look at them, how we react to them, if we can find a part of the situation to be gratoful for, we can change our feelings about it.

I believe we are here living our lives and living a life of happiness is the best thing we can achieve. I know when I used to blow my birthday candles out and I got to make a wish, my wish was always to be happy. I don't know what age I started with that wish but I do think it's the ultimate wish. If we are happy, we feel whole and complete and it has a contagious effect in many cases. In most situations or incidents when we deal with another person, if we are practicing a positive outlook and bring that to the interaction, the mood of the other person even though they may have been experiencing a feeling of negativity, can be lifted by our positive vibe. It's more difficult to have a negative interaction with a person who is obviously happy and in good spirits. Have you ever been confronted by an angry person who is intent on an argument and you smile and agree with them? It is surprising how you can take the wind right out of their sails, so to speak. Your unexpected response can instantly change their demeanor.

Deciding to be the most positive person in a situation can uplift others who are feeling down. Your energy can radiate to others and make them feel that all is well. We all have the power to shift from a negative to a positive force.

As I've said it's not something that we can do all the time. But it's a mindset worth cultivating. When things occur that would and do cause unhappiness, see the incident, accept the feelings related to it when it happens. Feeling it in the present time but not letting it define us. We can be happy people that deal with feelings related to things in our life which, when they occur, can bring feelings of unhappiness, sadness, and anger etc. That doesn't mean we need to be unhappy, sad or angry people or spend our precious time after the incident with those feelings.

We are all human. It is fine to have upset or even have a meltdown at times. Accepting what the feelings are in that moment. We all have times when we feel low or down. We don't need to be hard on ourselves for feeling like that. Having compassion as we would for someone else if they were not feeling ok. Being kind to ourselves. Accepting the feelings that go with difficult incidents but refocusing and moving on. Not making it a permanent place to be. Knowing that we can change the feelings with our own thoughts and actions moment by moment.

Don't relive any difficulty over and over, bringing It to the future. I've realised there are very few present moments in which we can't feel good. It is past and possible future events that cause us to have feelings of negativity.

The reader may think that it's not possible to get over a difficulty in the moment and then switch to being happy straight away. I agree! But if we are aware that we can bring ourselves to the now moment where that difficulty is not taking place at this time, we can focus on leaving the difficulty and lift how we feel. yes it will probably come back to our mind in ten minutes or an hour but with a present mindset we can focus our minds away from it and back to the present again. Find the positive aspects, be grateful for them and occupy our thoughts in the now moment. Look at the difficulty and decide whether it is within our control. Can we take steps to a solution, or is it outside of our control and there is no way we can fix it? We can give our concentration to something else and work on leaving the difficulty behind us for long periods and eventually permanently.

What goes on in our minds also effects our physical body and physical wellbeing. It is in our thoughts that the feelings which induce stress are created and there is a clear connection between stress causing illness and disease within our bodies. Our subconscious mind is alert to our thoughts all of the time. It is the part of the mind which stores the memory of how we feel about things we experience in our lives. Unresolved negative events that are stored in our subconscious can manifest physically, causing physical health problems over time. It could be from hurt, guilt, shame. Any negativity we carry with us does not serve us. What we practice grows stronger. We can choose to continue to feel guilt and shame over things in the past and make those feelings stronger with time or we can choose to use techniques like meditation, mindfulness, affirmations, gratitude and realise that we are not supposed to be perfect. Rather accept ourselves as we are. Love the unique individual you are and strive to practice this and have feelings of love and positivity. These feelings can grow stronger with time.

When we can't control what is happening around us we can always control how we react to it. This is where our power lies. Taking control of our response or reaction can change a situation to a positive or an indifferent one for us.

Each day is a new day for us all. Our mindset first thing

in the morning can determine how our day will be. I've mentioned starting the day with good expectations of how our day will go. Another positive way to start each day is with a feeling of gratitude, thankful for the day ahead. Since another day is another opportunity at life, no matter what has happened in the past, today can be a fresh start .

Acknowledging to ourselves as we get ready for the day, the things we have to be grateful for or writing a list before we start our day of things we are grateful for, even adding things that we are grateful to receive, is reiterating the expectation of them coming into our life. Gratitude is a powerful emotion and experiencing feelings of gratitude as we start and go about our day can bring about change in our life. It will keep our mind focused on the positive things we have and are experiencing in our life. Initially thoughts of gratitude brings to mind things of monetary value which we are grateful for. But the experience of gratitude is much more. It is an emotion which can strengthen relationships. It is about helping others and being helped. Feeling grateful boosts happiness and brings both physical and mental health benefits. Because of the connection between the mind and body, the feelings we evoke by being grateful have the power to shift negative attention away from our inner being and thus making our reality a more positive one.

Some people live their lives with feelings of 'poor me'. This is victim mentality. It can be brought on from experiences through their life of earlier incidents. People sometimes allow incidents to define them. Perhaps through illness, addiction or loss, they continue after recover to identify with this past mindset. We all experience things that are difficult. We need to accept that life can include hard times and can feel unfair. Prolonging the pain and suffering or using it as an excuse, only leads to more negative experiences. Acceptance is the key to dealing with difficulties that we cannot control and will alleviate the feelings of 'its not fair', 'why does this happen to me'? These feelings just brings further misery.

Gratitude for recovery and moving on from the feelings associated with past problems can give us a new perspective on how to view life. At any time we can make a decision to live from a place of gratitude, embracing life with a grateful outlook and sense of abundance in all experiences.

Because our feelings are so determined by thoughts and suggestions, writing and giving gratitude is positively suggesting to the mind that we are in the state of having received it. Being thankful for abundance, for good health, for perfect living conditions, for all we have and all we wish to have. Therefore suggesting to our mind it is already ours. Feel and act accordingly and through experiencing the feelings relevant to already having our desires in place and being grateful for them, as that changes so will our reality. A great way to get into the habit of showing gratitude and become aware of all the things we have to be grateful for, is to start writing a gratitude journal. Listing down a number of things each day that we are grateful for in our life, can also be helpful for lifting our mood at times when we are feeling low. It can also be useful to read back through such a journal, perhaps a year later to see how our lives and desires have changed ,in some cases maybe realising that the desires we held, would not have been a positive addition to our life. Instead what we received and how things unfolded in our lives was of greater benefit to us. Then giving gratitude for what comes to us in perfect timing in our lives.

The relationship with yourself must come first.

Self love is the starting point to sharing love.

Achieving happiness in our lives is I believe the ultimate goal. We hear regularly as people age about how they come to realise how fast the years go by. Every day is worth living to the full, and living our own life. I am very often surprised by the amount of time that people who have reached my age or older, live their lives restricted by other people's views or in some cases what they perceived to be other people's views. Whether it be a family member, work colleague, neighbors, friends they seem to value what others think or say above their own values and wishes. In some cases people think ,'oh I couldn't do that'. My children or parents or whoever in their life they have transferred their power to wouldn't like that. Or they think that would upset, annoyed others, so they live their lives not being true to their own values and wishes. Restricting themselves in the hope of keeping others happy and a general misguided flow of peace. But if we restrict ourselves to what we believe is other people's ideals for us, we are doing ourselves and them a disservice. We are individuals and we must be responsible for our own life. Just as other people cannot be responsible for our happiness we are not responsible for the happiness of others. We must all live our own lives learning from our mistakes and enjoying our achievements. To live to please other people will ultimately bring resentment and unease for one or both parties. Often people transfer their power without even realising it. It could be to a parent, spouse, partner, sibling or friend, even to our children and we can feel that we are ultimately living to keep others content. This can come about if a person in our life is more dominant or controlling or even someone we admire and convince ourselves that they know better than us. We love them and/or they love us and so we restrict ourselves to fit their values. They may suggest that limitations they put on us come from a place of love or concern. No one can live our lives better than we can ourselves. Taking responsibility for our own life, putting ourselves first is not a selfish act.

It is the way to a fulfilling life and if we are not fulfilled and feeling whole we cannot be a positive family member or friend to any one else. It is our responsibility to fill our lives with our desires, it is not possible to pour from an empty cup and so it is actually a selfless act, to put our own happiness and desires first. Living our life to our own needs and values, is taking responsibility for ourselves .

'He \ she loves themselves' was, when I was growing up a criticism of someone. I think times are changing in that regard. But not in all cases. Loving yourself is an achievement and not one everyone finds easy. People tend to criticize themselves or put conditions and time lines on themselves and things in their lives. Eg. I will be happy when I lose weight or when I get my new house or when I have a baby and so on. However accepting that things in our life will happen when the time is right, having gratitude and believing that all will be well, keeping our thoughts and mindset on the positive aspects of our life is the recipe for happiness.

To be responsible for our life and have peace of mind is to decide we do not need approval from others or prove ourselves in situations. We do not need to convince people of our thinking or our side of the story and accept the same of them. What is most important is within us. That which feels right and true to ourselves. The experiences that feel good. If we focus on our own truths we will project positivity to others and have no need to look for validation in our lives.

Loving ourselves and putting ourselves first does not mean that we cannot be of service to the people around us. Some people might be in a position that they run a house and take care of the whole families needs. Or perhaps spend a great deal of time taking care of vulnerable or sick people as a volunteer. In the situation where this is fulfilling to them, this is self love. In a situation where they feel the choice is not theirs and they resent doing it, this is not serving them. In this type of situation, it is their responsibility to themselves to take account of and change the situation. Doing things in life that we are not happy about doing, because we feel it is expected of us, will bring feelings of resentment into our life, this is an negative emotion. It's up to us to take responsibility for ourselves and change the situation. keeping negative emotions out of our life is only possible by our own actions in situations that we are unhappy with.

Self love is being true to our self and living the life we deserve, when we have difficulty loving our self we often find our self in situations we resent and find it hard to change as we believe that we do not deserve better.

Self criticism is one of the most destructive components that keeps us from loving our self, and it is widespread in conversations and thoughts. I can't, I'm too this or that, I wish I was, if I only could, not me. So many times in so many ways we put ourselves down. We tell ourselves we are not good enough, criticize our image, our ability, our lives, our achievements. These are all affirmations but they are negative affirmations. Just like the positive ones I spoke of earlier, the more we say them, accept the feelings and emotions they evoke, the more they become part of our reality. We live by them and they effect how we feel about ourselves and how we behave. They determine our self worth and make the difference in our lives between being loving to ourselves or putting others first and living with regret and resentment. Feeling undeserving and unworthy of a happy life is unconsciously resisting growth and positive change in our life. Forgiving ourselves with compassion and accepting that we are all different and are all as worthy as each other. We all make mistakes in life, we are here to learn and grow and live fulfilling lives loving ourselves and others, that is the key. The most important person for us to love is ourselves, only then can we love others.

Using the analogy of a garden. To consider whether we are living a life that is serving us well. We can imagine 6 or more flower pots each containing a part of our life. In one perhaps we have planted a relationship or marriage, in the next our children and family. The third one contains our friends, the next one our work and in another our hobbies, maybe pets, travel, relaxation, all the different components of a happy life. All areas of our life that we like to give time to. Our garden is blossoming. But at some point maybe one or two plants leave our life. We lose our job or our children leave home. There will always be changes in our lives. This is why it's important to plant many plant pots in the garden. Because if one goes, we have an empty space, but our garden can still blossom with all the other plants. We still have many things to enjoy in our life. We can make the mistake of living life with our complete focus on one plant pot. Tending to this one plant and giving all our attention and time to it. For some people that can be work or perhaps their children, maybe their relationship. With the result if this one thing leaves their life they feel they have nothing else. It is part of self love to live a balanced life. Doing the things we enjoy and making time for different experiences in our life, so that a full and varied garden of plant pots thrive.

Choosing to be happy and enjoying positive feelings more of the time is a choice. We all have difficulties to deal with in life. However, purpose and meaning ,different experiences, balance, and connections with others can all assist in creating a happy life.

When coming from a place of love and trying to help a friend who is experiencing difficulty in their life, to empathise with them is love. However in the process, taking on the difficulty ourselves, with the result that we diminish our own positive feelings to help them feel better is serving no one well. Taking on another's energy can have the effect of depleting our own. Being true to our own inner feelings does not lessen the help we can offer. We do not need to distinguish our own light, to be of service to others.

Love is a powerful emotion, and living from a place of love is an inside job. We must accept that we are worthy and have compassion for ourselves. Don't beat ourselves up when things go wrong or we have a bad day. Decide that guilt and blame are destructive in our life, whether to ourselves or others and serve no purpose. Create a mindset of kindness, care and being true to ourselves and our needs. When we deliberately decide that these are the values we are going to live with in our life, we will express ourselves differently and these values will be automatically extended to other people too. Because when we feel good about ourselves we have no interest in expressing negativity to others. We are happy and exude feelings of positivity to others as we interact. Have you noticed when you get the sharp end of someone's tongue, it is generally because they are not feeling good and release their anger onto others? It works the other way too. Happy people radiate joy, love and kindness so spending our time on our own happiness will have a contagious affect.

I've said earlier that I believe living in a state of happiness is the ultimate goal in life. Being in alignment with the universal energy, otherwise described as being in a high vibration is the state we need to aspire to. It is a state of believing that we are here in physical form but that our energy is part of a universal energy. This I refer to as source energy. When we start to consider our thoughts and how our minds are so intrinsic to our feelings, it leads to more questioning about life and whether we are getting the most from it. Spiritual awareness is where we are lead when the questions I referred to at the beginning of this book are asked. Whether we are all connected and how to live a complete and satisfying life?

Spirituality suggests there is more to life than what we experience on a physical level. It maintains there is a greater power which connects us to each other and also to a universal power. It's a belief in something beyond our physical being. In essence a journey in life towards a greater awareness. The experience of spirituality can be different and varied for people. It is a realisation that there is more than what we experience physically. For people living a spiritual life it gives a sense of meaning to life. It offers a sense of connection to source, nature and all humanity. It involves experiencing compassion for others, in the belief that we are all connected, so a deepening understanding and empathy for others can be gained. We can find happiness beyond our possessions or material belongings and any external factors.

Spirituality is something I believe that comes through awareness. It is an individual experience. It doesn't come with a set of rules. It is more of a personal journey, finding purpose and developing a greater, more positive outlook on life.

Exploring it can offer answers to question about the meaning of life and our purpose in being here. Belief in a universal connection brings feelings of well being, less stress and can ultimately create a trust in life and the life path we are on, believing that all is unfolding as it is meant to and in the perfect timing in our life. Through this type of belief and faith, the fear of death can be greatly diminished. The belief in a connection to source energy offers a trust in what is unfolding while we are experiencing life in our physical bodies and beyond with our non physical being.

Practicing meditation and mindfulness, and becoming

aware when we are living in the present moment is often the start of self discovery and spiritual awakening. The positive feelings we start to experience will lead to wanting greater insight into living a happy fulfilling life. We realise it is available to us and start the journey to find out and enjoy more in our lives.

So where to start? I have covered the starting points of living a happy life.

1 Starting our day, deliberately deciding it will be a good day

2 Listing the things in our life we are grateful for

3 Speaking or writing positive affirmations about ourselves and our world

4 Taking responsibility for our life and what happens in it

5 Keeping our thoughts in the present as much as possible and enjoy what we focus on at that time

6 Practice meditation \mindfulness \yoga

7 Love ourselves and do what we love.

8 Reframe negative thoughts.

9 Knowing we don't need the approval of others. Only our own.

10 Living from a place of love.

Love is the universal connection.

We came here to live in love.

We are spiritual beings in a physical body. We are part
of a universal energy. We came to experience a fulfilling
life in our physical body. Love is the reality of our reason
for living. we are much more than our bodies we have
a mind and a consciousness and are connected to the
source energy we came from. I call it source, although it
is known by many other names. Higher power, light of the
world. It is unimportant what it is called it is the energy
that we are all connected to. As I referred to earlier, it is
the believe we hold when we are living life conscious of
our universal connection. It is love. We came from it to live
and experience a life of love. Many worldly influences as
we grow and live our lives cause us to shift from living lives
of love to lives of fear. We were born with love and learned
fear. Everything is defined by love or fear. Our thoughts,
words and actions are love or fear based. Fear is a lack of
trust in ourselves and the universal energy that we are part
of. If we love ourselves and others, we have no reason to be
fearful. We are all connected, we breathe the same air, live
in the same world in our physical bodies and have the same
needs. Perfect health, nourishment and to feel love and give
love. The only separation is our physical beings, beyond
that we are connected. If we accept this and believe that
this is our desire and birthright when we are born then we
realise that all we need is already within us. We can then
live a life of love and trust and have no need to be fearful of
how our life unfolds. Accept, that with belief in ourselves,
everything will work out perfectly and in perfect timing.
Straying from a path of love with thoughts, words or actions
is what is disruptive and destructive in our lives. All we need
is within us. Living from this mindset will bring peace of
mind.

To live our lives from a place of love is to be conscious of
our thoughts, words and actions. These have the power
to make our reality positive or negative. What comes
to mind when you hear the word spiritual? Sometimes

religion and spirituality can be confused, we can practice religion and live a spiritual life, or live a spiritual life without being religious. Often religious traditions are centered on worshiping a higher power. However the teachings can involve a fear based consequence on the subject of how we live our lives and worship the higher power. Fear based teachings are not part of the spiritual path. Spirituality is an awareness of the universal energy we all share. To live in awareness on a spiritual path is to believe that we are all connected to each other and are part of Source. It is to live from a place of love without fear, with all creation and all humanity as one. All the good and evil in the world, all humanity, creatures and nature are all part of that energy and it effects us all. So the more positivity and love that is present the better for us all as we are all part of the same universal energy. To put it another way, how we treat others is how we treat ourselves as we are all part of the same universal energy. Whatever we put out into the world becomes part of that universal energy. Every interaction we have with another comes from love or fear. A spiritual life is to experience living when we do not partake in the criticism of others or get any satisfaction from others mistakes or misfortunes. To feel only positive feelings towards others, even people that we feel wronged by. To show love to another, not with the expectation of a pat on the back or a reward from them. The reward being a positive interaction for all. To add positivity to the universal energy.

To get no satisfaction from speaking and relaying negative news or incidents in our life and the world in general is to live in love with others. It is to be aligned with source, one does not work without the other, we are all one. All part of the same universal energy.

We as humans have all learned the behavior, to be judgmental, jealous, critical, argumentative and there are many more negative traits we exhibit. If we can accept all, we can live in the state of love that we have come from. When we become conscious of this, and live in the knowledge that we are part of source and not alone, but connected to a source of love which can be relied upon, we can then remove fear from our lives. Becoming aware of our thoughts and working on staying present, perhaps though meditation or mindfulness we can then accept that it is only the present moment at any time we can live. Accepting that it is our thoughts that determine how we feel and we do not need to alter the actions of others. When we accept this it can assist us in giving up traits like judgment, criticism and comparisons with others .We can experience a feeling of wholeness within ourselves. It is from a place of dissatisfaction with our own lives that prevents us from showing love to others. Whatever we radiate to others is what is within us. To send out love we must have a loving mindset and we are the only one capable and responsible for obtaining that for ourselves.

How would it feel to not be in fear of anything ? To believe that we are always connected to the source of love that we came from. When we live from that perspective then even when the negativity that is constantly brought into your life from outside sources such as fears of terrorists, illness, poverty and death, no longer impacts on our feelings. Our consciousness knows that there is nothing to fear and so we live from a place of love. As such, our connection to source is love not fear. The life we experience in our physical body is connected to the universal energy that we came from. By living in love and being aligned with the source we came from, there is no need to experience fear for our future. The more we practice living in love, the more we will have alignment with source. Alignment with source comes from positive energy and good feelings. Whatever we can do in our lives to obtain positive, loving feelings within, increases our alignment with source. It can be achieved in different ways. For some it can be through meditation, for others walking in nature or sitting on a beach enjoying the sun. Raising feelings of love for yourself and others is the path to alignment with source.

We are constantly surrounded by information coming from many media sources that is fear based and evokes fear in our society. It is quite amazing when you become aware of how many negative, fearful incidents we are presented with and absorb on a daily basis. It is common for a complete news bulletin to be fear filled from start to finish. If we constantly absorb this, it can cause us to live from a place of fear. Which in turn causes us to look outside ourselves for help. We look to others to save us from these disasters which have been brought to our attention. In many cases these things will not be a direct threat to us. Whether it is health scares, financial doom or terrorism the result is that we are giving our power away. We are handing responsibility for our lives over to someone else to fix or save us. The more we do this the more we give responsibility for our lives and our happiness to others. We fail to accept we are the ones responsible for our own lives. We disregard the connection we have to the source of love that we are created from and can be aligned with. As I've said and it is worth saying again, fear is a lack of trust in ourselves.

To be in alignment with source is to live a life of love without fear. Coming from love will always be acting in the right way without fear of consequences. It is coming from within ourselves owning our power and taking responsibility for our own lives. Knowing that our actions are true and our values are based in love.

Positive emotions come from love, negative emotions from fear.

Love is positive. It is kind and caring. It motivate and

encourages. It is patient, accepting and it is contagious.

Fear is negative. It is reactive, hurtful, dismissive, frightening, controlling and it is also contagious.

Contagion is the only one on both lists. Love and fear can be spread as easily as each other. The more people that choose love, the more positivity that will be experienced globally.

The only place that fear exists is in the mind. It is an emotion that is linked to our survival. It is the reaction to a threat to our wellbeing and the feelings it evokes are stored in our subconscious and recalled by those same feelings in the future. But in most cases we are creating fear in our minds from situations that are not present treats at all. Negative thoughts from suggestions are often exaggerated and are not part of our actual life unless we allow it. Our physical bodies react to suggestions, as mine did when I was giving birth to my son. So suggestions we absorb of fear can cause negative physical reactions in our bodies. None of us know what the future holds. We only have the present moment at any time. Accepting and embracing this is very liberating. Knowing that we cannot control situations that may occur in the future but rather living with a positive expectation of the future. Loving the present moment results in love and positivity radiating out from us, what radiate out from us will come back to us. This is then what we can expect in our lives.

Just as happiness is an inside job living from love is also an inside job. It is taking responsibility for our own life. We have all been blessed with a different combination of gifts, talents, passions and the experiences we have are ours. We are all unique, but part of a universal energy. We are all as worthy as each other. We are all part of the one and we are all needed. If we accept this as true, it is difficult to understand why there is so much conflict in the world. We have the opportunity as we live a life of love to change not only our own experiences, but by sharing this to change experiences globally for the better .

All the things I have spoken of can not be put in place to change our mindset in an instant. Rather it is a process it is like any life style change we are interested in adopting. It starts with awareness and a desire for a happier life. We all deal with different challenges going through life. Living a life based on the principals of remaining in the moment, coming from a place of love, for ourselves and others, giving rather then wanting and having a trust in life, this will be the cornerstone of experiencing a happier reality. To live a life of love, forgiveness, patience and acceptance takes a great deal of inner work. It is a journey. We can wander off the path and lose our way sometimes. But the path is always there and we can return to it at any time without feelings of guilt or failure. We may be just out of alignment for a time but we can always choose to go within and reconnect with source. Being aware of what we are contributing to the universal energy is the way to enlightenment and happiness.

That is not to say that challenging times will not affect us. When we need to deal with difficulties and our mood drops and we feel the emotions that we associate with negativity this is normal. It's about being true to ourselves and what we are experiencing and the real emotions associated with it. Accepting the feelings that are relevant to what is happening for us at any time. Accepting them, does not mean we have lost our connection to source. We must not beat ourselves up when we are not in top form. We should experience all the emotions of what is happening in our lives at any particular time. However with a mindset that at any time there is only that moment to deal with. If we are coming from a place of love we are doing the right thing.

We must love ourselves through difficult times, even when we are experiencing negative emotions. Whatever it is we are dealing with we must allow ourselves the time we need to get through it. With an acceptance that this is what we need to be true to the unique individual we are and are deserving of our feelings. That will give us an assurance and the confidence to deal with challenges when they occur in our lives.

When we face challenges, whether health, loss, disappointments, consider are they sent to interrupt our lives, or are they a wake up call to change something? Has our life, become out of balance? Are we experiencing enough joy? Or are we overloading our lives with duty and being hard on ourselves? How are we spending our time? Are we absorbing fear and negativity? These are the questions we need to ask ourselves. When our lives are out of balance, the stress we experience can manifest in our physical reality.

Perhaps at this stage, the reader is asking, where do we start with these changes to lead to a more fulfilling life? Living a very busy life and considering these life style changes in the search of a more fulfilling and happier life, can seem like adding further stress and possible feelings of failure. But it can happen in small steps simply by having awareness as we go about our lives. Our feelings are the perfect monitor to alignment with source. Any positive changes that we make can lead to the motivation to continue.

As I have said, we are all different, we are all on our own life path. Every experience we have is different from another's. There may be similarities with our experiences on life's journey. But each of us are unique and as such our experiences are too. So whatever steps we take to change our life, can only be decided by ourselves. Others may help with advice or suggestions, but they can not know better than we do ourselves. Our feelings can determine what is right or wrong for our own life no one else can do the journey for us. So whatever way, or pace we take, it is an individual journey for each of us. We decide why, when, how we wish to live. Knowing what feels good or bad in each situation is what will help us to achieve the reality we want.

I believe by an awareness of the connection between ourselves and the source that we came from and we are always connected to, is the basis of leading a fulfilling life. There can be many challenges in the modern world we live in today to overcome. Living with a belief in our connection to source can certainly take the pressure off. It is the belief in a connection to all and a knowing that we are all as worthy as each other. Being aware of our connection to source offers a reassurance and trust in difficult times. There isn't one way or a rule book to living life. It is an individual experience and can differ for us all because it comes from within ourselves. There are lots of different aspects but many are common to people who are living in awareness of the universal connection, or are starting to make it part of their day to day lives. It often starts with the journey of self discovery and a need to try to get more from life. To find purpose and meaning in life. Taking stock of our current believes. When we reflect on questions we have about life without pressure to find the answers, just continuing to live and enjoy what we are doing, that is often when answers can present themselves from within. We can get comfortable relying on our gut feelings.

Awareness of the universal connection allows compassion for ourselves and others as we are all part of the human experience and we are all here to enjoy it. Allowing ourselves to love, without judgement and to live in a state of acceptance with what we cannot change or control.

Believing all is well in our world. Connecting to nature and spending time outdoors where we can become grounded and be part of the energy of that space. Feeding our mind and body, with wholesome thoughts and healthy food. Clearing our mind and possibly the space we inhabit to aid clarity of thought. These are all steps which we can adopt as part of our lives. These steps along with ones that I have already shared in the book, like meditation, mindfulness, yoga, gratitude, love, the list could go on, are all positive steps to a happier and more fulfilling life .The intention on a spiritual path is to find fulfillment in life and to share it as we interact with others. We can bring an awareness to others, who simply recognise something positive about our lives and experiences and have a desire to discover more and become part of the connection and love we experience.

All the experiences, I have written about and covered in this book are components to living with happiness and fulfillment. However to sum it up and put it into just three words to live, and enjoy our lives by ...

Connection --------------------Love ------------------Faith .

Affirmations

Gratitude

A note from the author.

I was born in Dublin, Ireland in 1963. I lived there most of my life. Travel is something I enjoy, and am now based in southern Spain. I have enjoyed a blessed life in a caring family with loving parents. I've always been fortunate to have a positive outlook, which I in part attribute to my dad, who's positive outlook and good humor are over present . My work life has been varied. I ran my own retail business for a number of years. I am very much a people person, so enjoyed the interaction with people that all my work roles involved. Since my teenage years, I have written short stories and in latter years that turned more to journaling, resulting in my interest of self development which lead me to study relevant courses online. That is how this book came to be. My wish is that it has given you inspiration to reflect on the reality you are experiencing. If change is something that you desire, go within yourself and start making it happen. Life is short, is a regularly used phase, so don't let it pass, without experiencing the joy.

I have very much enjoyed writing this book. For me writing and reading over it, has kept these beliefs in the forefront of my mind. I want to express my gratitude to my good friend, Allison Greene who kindly assisted me during the process with the grammar, punctuation and editing. Which is not my forte but I'm pleased to say I have learned a bit through the process. I also want to extend thanks to my friend Deirdre Flannery for her work on bringing my idea for the cover to life.